Healthy living: The Connection Between Exercise and Mental Health

By

Martha Z. Lee

Table of Content

Introduction

A man by the name of John used to live in the busy metropolis of Metropolis, but he was always caught up in the turmoil of his hectic and demanding life. His days as a corporate executive were dominated by pinging emails nonstop, endless meetings, and strict deadlines. He was carrying a lot of responsibility, and it was becoming more and more obvious how this was affecting his mental health.

While John was navigating the concrete jungle one day, he happened upon a small fitness studio tucked away between the tall skyscrapers. He chose to enroll in the "Mindful Movement" class because it piqued his interest and offered a brief reprieve from the chaos of his regular life.

The instructor, a cheerful woman named Sarah, smiled warmly to greet John. He had no idea that this random meeting would serve as the impetus for a drastic change in his physical and mental well-being.

John experienced the joy of reestablishing a connection with his body and breath as he immersed himself in the world of mindful movement. The rhythmic movements and gentle yoga poses turned into a haven where he could temporarily stop his mind's incessant chatter. Sensing John's journey, Sarah highlighted the release of endorphins and the calming effect on the nervous system as she discussed the complex relationship between exercise and mental health.

As the days stretched into weeks, John made a commitment to consistent exercise—not just as a habit, but as a vital component of his mental health. The executive, who had been under stress, found comfort in just moving his body. He found solace in the yoga studio, where he could clearly feel the link between physical and mental well-being.

John noticed a change in himself gradually but definitely. In the midst of chaos, he was able to find clarity as the stress fog lifted. In addition to building up his physical strength, the exercise proved to be an effective means of reducing stress, anxiety, and even the sporadic episodes of depression.

Encouraged by his newfound knowledge of the link between physical activity and mental well-being, John started telling friends and coworkers about his experience. Others were motivated by his journey to investigate the ways in which physical activity can support mental health.

A small but notable change was observed in Metropolis as more people began to prioritize exercising for their mental health. Joggers crowded the parks, businesses adopted wellness initiatives, and abandoned gym memberships turned into symbols of self-care.

John's story turned into a ray of hope, demonstrating the healing potential of acknowledging and fostering the link between physical activity and mental well-being. In the midst of the tall skyscrapers and the bustling city, a community rose up, one that recognized the beautiful interdependence of a healthy body and mind rather than their mutual exclusion.

In a world where life seems to move at an unstoppable pace, the significance of mental health has become paramount. "The Connection Between Exercise and Mental Health" is more than just a book; it's an invitation to delve into the life-changing relationship between exercise and mental toughness. Three essential components serve as our road map as we set out to explore the deep connection between physical activity and mental well-being.

Mental Health as a Priority: Our overall well-being is greatly impacted by our mental health, which is no longer a minor concern in the busyness of our daily lives. We'll start by reviewing the current status of mental health, recognizing its impact on society, its prevalence, and the necessity of using holistic approaches. This lays the groundwork for a deeper comprehension of how putting mental health first can result in a life that is more balanced and fulfilling.

Exercise as a Dynamic Intervention: Our exploration goes beyond traditional ideas of exercise and goes beyond the pursuit of physical fitness alone. We'll explore the complex ways that physical activity functions as a dynamic mental health intervention. We'll delve into the science underlying the mood-boosting effects of exercise, from the production of endorphins to the alterations in brain physiology. This section provides guidance on utilizing physical activity as a proactive, empowering decision for mental well-being, rather than just as a routine.

Unveiling the Science: We sort through the scientific details and simplify the mysterious relationship between exercise and mental health. As we examine how exercise affects neurotransmitters, modifies the structure of the brain, and enhances cognitive function, neurobiology takes center stage. We'll make the connections, arming you with strong research evidence and a thorough grasp of the physiological and psychological processes that underpin exercise's effectiveness as a mental health enhancer.

"The Connection Between Exercise and Mental Health" is a thorough investigation that provides direction, wisdom, and useful information. This book is a road map to realizing the potential in your body and mind, whether you're looking for strategies to reduce stress, overcome obstacles, or improve your general quality of life. Come along on this exploratory journey with us, where the act of moving itself can cause a profound transformation. Let's clear the path to a happier, healthier, and more resilient life together.

Chapter I
The State of Mental Health

The condition of mental health has become a crucial thread in the complex tapestry of human existence, impacting the very fabric of our existence. This chapter deconstructs the current state of mental health, illuminating the incidence of mental health disorders, their significant social impact, and the pressing need for all-encompassing strategies to address these problems.

1. Statistics on the Prevalence of Mental Health Disorders:

The brutal reality is that mental health issues are widespread and cut across social, cultural, and geographic divides. Roughly one in four people will at some point in their lives experience a mental health disorder, according to recent global health surveys. Particularly, anxiety and depression have spread like silent epidemics, impacting millions of people globally. These figures highlight how urgent it is to address mental health problems and acknowledge that they are a common human experience.

2. The Societal Impact of Mental Health Issues:

Beyond personal hardships, mental health problems have a significant impact on society. There are noticeable knock-on effects, ranging from strained personal relationships to decreased workplace productivity. Issues related to mental health have a significant impact on the worldwide disease burden, resulting in extensive social and economic ramifications. The influence on society is not limited to the person with the illness; it also affects families, communities, and establishments. Because mental health issues are often silent, people tend to undervalue their impact, which perpetuates a widespread underestimation of the problem's severity.

3. The Need for Holistic Approaches to Mental Health:

Traditionally, mental health treatments have been divided into distinct areas, with the main goal being to reduce symptoms with medicine or counseling. But a paradigm shift is necessary in light of our expanding understanding of mental health as a complex and interrelated component of overall well- being. Holistic approaches take into account the larger context in which mental health is situated in addition to the symptoms. This includes social relationships, lifestyle choices, physical health, and—most importantly—the function that exercise plays in preserving and reestablishing mental balance.

The shortcomings of isolated therapies highlight the necessity of an all-encompassing framework that acknowledges the complex interactions between the body and mind. Holistic approaches to mental health recognize the significance of elements like exercise, stress reduction, sleep, and nutrition. In light of this, investigating the relationship between physical activity and mental health seems like a promising way to advance overall wellbeing.

Understanding the urgency of taking a more inclusive and integrated approach to mental health is vital as we set out on this journey. We can address the complex issues that mental health poses in a more compassionate and efficient manner by acknowledging the impact that mental health disorders have on society, appreciating how common they are, and adopting holistic approaches. The next few chapters will go into greater detail about exercise's crucial role in this all-encompassing approach and how it can change the mental health landscape.

Chapter II
Understanding Exercise as a Mental Health Intervention

Few interventions have the transformative power that exercise has over our mental health when it comes to holistic well-being. This chapter explores the complex psychological mechanisms that underlie the strong correlation between exercise and mental health in an effort to piece together the many advantages that physical activity bestows upon our psychological well-being.

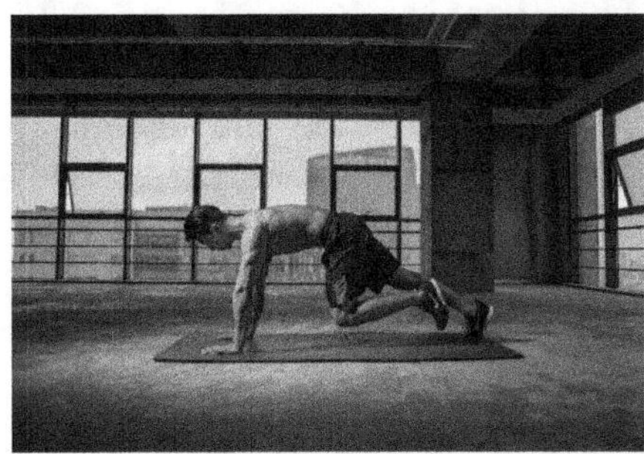

Overview of the Benefits of Exercise on Mental Well-being

Exercise has many advantages that go far beyond the physical and into the complex depths of our mental and emotional health. Regular physical activity triggers a series of beneficial effects that impact mood, cognitive function, and mental health in general.

Release of Endorphins and their Impact on Mood- The release of endorphins, sometimes known as the body's natural mood enhancers, is central to the exercise-mood relationship. These neurotransmitters produce feelings of euphoria and wellbeing in addition to acting as pain modulators. Exercise releases a burst of endorphins that balance out the negative effects of stress and anxiety by fostering a deep sense of positivity.

Reduction of Stress Hormones through Physical Activity- Exercise reduces the effects of the body's stress response and is a powerful stress reliever. Physical activity regulates the release of cortisol, which is the main hormone released during stress. People who exercise successfully regulate their levels of stress hormones, which results in a more balanced and tranquil state of mind.

Improvement of Sleep Patterns and their Role in Mental Health- Sleep is essential for mental health and is closely related to regular physical activity. Exercise is essential for controlling sleep patterns in addition to improving the quality of sleep. Sleep's restorative qualities support mental clarity, emotional stability, and cognitive performance.

Examination of the Psychological Mechanisms Behind Exercise and Mental Health

Beyond its obvious effects on stress and mood, exercise has a deeper connection to mental health. Physical activity promotes holistic well-being, which is facilitated by a complex interplay of psychological mechanisms beneath the physiological changes.

Neurotransmitter Regulation- Serotonin and dopamine are two neurotransmitters that are significantly impacted by exercise. Known as the "feel-good" neurotransmitter, serotonin is an essential neurotransmitter that regulates mood and emotional health. Dopamine, on the other hand, is linked to pleasure and reward, which helps explain why engaging in physical activity makes one feel motivated and accomplished.

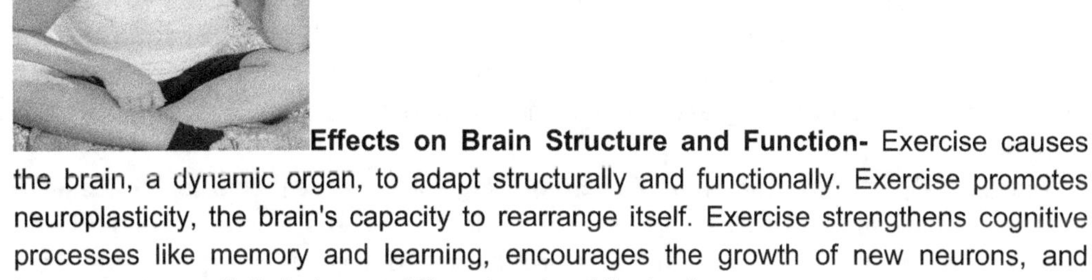

Effects on Brain Structure and Function- Exercise causes the brain, a dynamic organ, to adapt structurally and functionally. Exercise promotes neuroplasticity, the brain's capacity to rearrange itself. Exercise strengthens cognitive processes like memory and learning, encourages the growth of new neurons, and improves connectivity between different parts of the brain.

We will dive deeper into the science underlying the relationship between exercise and mental health in the upcoming chapters. We will examine the neurobiological alterations that transpire during physical activity, bolstered by persuasive case studies and research outcomes that shed light on the significant influence that physical activity can have on our mental health. Exercise is more than just a physical activity; as we explore the nuances of this relationship, it becomes clear that it is a potent intervention for promoting and maintaining our mental health.

Chapter III
The Science Behind the Connection

We now focus on the complex interactions between the body and brain in our investigation of the profound relationship between physical activity and mental health. By delving into the neurobiological alterations that occur during exercise and presenting gripping case studies and research findings that highlight the significant influence of physical activity on our mental health, this chapter aims to shed light on the science underlying this dynamic relationship.

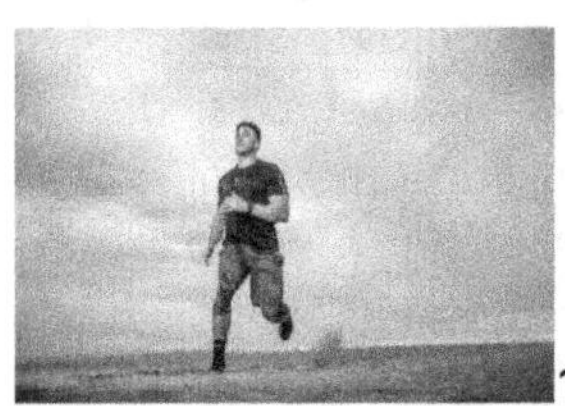

1. Exploration of Neurobiological Changes During Exercise

Exercise activates the human brain, which is a finely tuned network of neurons and neurotransmitters that experiences a symphony of changes. People who exercise experience a series of neurobiological processes that all work together to improve mental health.

Impact on Neurotransmitters such as Serotonin and Dopamine- Serotonin and dopamine in particular are powerful neurotransmitter modulators that are influenced by exercise. Elevated serotonin synthesis and release are linked to mood regulation and emotional health. Increased dopamine levels also reinforce the positive association between physical activity and feelings of reward and pleasure.

Effects on Brain Structure and Function- Regular exercise helps to harness the brain's neuroplasticity. The stimulation of neurotrophic factors, such as brain-derived neurotrophic factor (BDNF), aids in the development and maintenance of neurons. As a result, the brain undergoes structural alterations, including an increase in gray matter volume in areas linked to cognitive and emotional regulation.

Influence on Stress Response and Cortisol Regulation- Exercise influences the body's reaction to stressors by acting as a natural stress buffer. Physical activity has the ability to modulate the primary stress hormone, cortisol. This helps create a more robust stress response system in addition to lessening the negative effects of chronic stress.

2. The Link Between Exercise and Mental Health:

There is strong confirmation to support the compelling relationship between exercise and mental health, including numerous case studies and substantial research that highlight the positive effects of physical activity.

Depression and Anxiety- Exercise has been shown in numerous studies to be effective in reducing symptoms of anxiety and depression. The evidence continuously shows that regular physical activity can be just as beneficial as conventional therapeutic interventions in reducing symptoms and preventing relapse, from randomized controlled trials to longitudinal studies.

Cognitive Function and Memory- Studies have demonstrated how exercise improves memory and cognitive function. In addition to improving executive skills like focus and decision-making, exercise stimulates the growth of new neurons in the hippocampus, an area vital to memory consolidation. This process is known as neurogenesis.

Sleep Quality and Mental Well-being- It is commonly known that exercise improves the quality of sleep. Studies show that sleeping longer and having a more restorative sleep cycle are benefits of regular physical activity, in addition to increasing sleep duration. Since sleep is essential for both emotional control and cognitive function, the effects on mental health are significant.

It's becoming more and more clear as we explore the scientific literature on the relationship between exercise and mental health that the advantages go well beyond the realm of the body. Exercise's neurobiological effects, along with the strong evidence from research and case studies, highlight the effectiveness of physical activity as a comprehensive intervention for mental health. We will explore the various types of exercise and their unique benefits for mental health in more detail in the upcoming chapters, revealing the subtle ways that various modalities support our psychological well-being.

Chapter IV
Types of Exercise and Their Mental Health Benefits

As we investigate the mutually beneficial relationship between physical activity and mental health, it becomes clear that not all physical activities have the same psychological effects. This chapter explores the variety of exercise modalities, each providing a special set of advantages for mental health. We'll cover a wide range of topics, including the energizing effects of aerobic exercise on mood, the strengthening effect of strength training on mental resilience, and the stress-relieving properties of mind-body activities like yoga and tai chi. We will also emphasize how important it is to match personal preferences with the exercise of choice, acknowledging the close relationship between enjoyment on a personal level and long-term mental health benefits.

1. Aerobic Exercises and Their Impact on Mood:

Aerobic workouts have become well-known for their ability to significantly improve mood. They are defined by prolonged, rhythmic activities that raise the heart rate. Running, cycling, and swimming all have a rhythmic quality that encourages the body's natural mood enhancers, endorphins, to be released. Frequent aerobic exercises have been shown to enhance self-esteem, lessen anxiety and depression symptoms, and provide a sense of accomplishment.

2. Strength Training and Its Influence on Mental Resilience:

Strength training not only helps with physical change but also develops mental toughness. Resistance training, which involves gradually increasing the body's level of difficulty, promotes resilience, discipline, and resolve. People frequently experience a corresponding rise in mental toughness when they observe the observable gains in strength and endurance; this leads to higher levels of self-efficacy and a more resilient mindset when faced with obstacles in life.

3. Mind-Body Exercises (e.g., Yoga, Tai Chi) and Their Role in Stress Reduction:

Exercises for the mind and body, like yoga and tai chi, provide a comprehensive approach to mental and physical health. These techniques combine breathing, movement, and awareness to produce a calming combination that mitigates the negative effects of stress. Together with the soft, flowing movements, the intentional attention to the present moment triggers a relaxation response in the neurological system, lowering cortisol levels and fostering a deep sense of balance and tranquility.

4. The Importance of Finding the Right Exercise for Individual Preferences:

Exercise has several, scientifically proven advantages for mental health, but achieving these benefits depends on personal inclination. There is no one-size-fits-all approach to mental health. It requires that the workout modality selected be in line with individual inclinations and interests. The exercise that is selected should speak to the person personally, whether it is the energizing rush of a morning run, the empowering sense of lifting weights, or the meditative serenity of a yoga session.

Recognizing and honoring personal preferences when it comes to exercise improves mental health outcomes in addition to increasing commitment to physical activity. Exercise regimens that are customized to an individual's interests, objectives, and physical capabilities promote a long-lasting and pleasurable approach to wellbeing.

It's evident as we explore the variety of exercise modalities in this chapter that everyone can find a kind of physical activity that not only supports their physical health but also fosters their mental and emotional well-being. We will examine the psychological and preventive benefits of exercise for mental health in the upcoming chapters, as well as how these activities can be incorporated into daily routines and treatment plans for the best possible outcome.

Chapter V
Exercise as a Preventive and Therapeutic Tool

Exercise plays a dual role in the complex relationship between mental health and physical activity. It serves as a preventive measure as well as a therapeutic tool. This chapter explores the dual nature of exercise, including its potential to prevent mental health disorders, its incorporation into treatment plans that are comprehensive, and the subtle difficulties and factors that must be taken into account when putting exercise interventions for mental health into practice.

Examining Exercise as a Preventive Measure Against Mental Health Disorders

A robust mental health framework's foundation is prevention, and exercise is a powerful ally in this effort. Recent research indicates that engaging in regular physical activity provides a strong protective effect against the emergence of a number of mental health conditions. Exercise builds emotional resilience and lessens the effects of stressors, acting as a preventative measure against the development of disorders like depression and anxiety. Exercise becomes a proactive investment in long-term mental health by promoting a resilient mind-body connection.

Integration of Exercise into Mental Health Treatment Plans

Exercise is not just for prevention; it is a seamless part of treatment plans for mental health issues. Physical activity's all-encompassing advantages enhance conventional therapeutic approaches and offer a comprehensive strategy for mental health. Including exercise in treatment plans improves the overall effectiveness of interventions, including medication and cognitive-behavioral therapies. Exercise has proven to be a flexible and encouraging part of mental health treatment, whether used as an independent therapeutic tool or as an additional measure.

Challenges and Considerations in Implementing Exercise Interventions

Exercise has been shown to have significant positive effects on mental health, but putting these benefits into practice can present certain difficulties. It is imperative to comprehend and tackle these obstacles in order to maximize the efficacy of exercise-based interventions.

1. Individual Variability and Preferences- It's critical to acknowledge that people differ in their physical capacities, tastes, and comfort levels when it comes to exercise. Customizing interventions to meet the preferences of each individual increases adherence and optimizes the positive effects on mental health.

2. Motivation and Adherence- Motivation is necessary to maintain a regular exercise regimen, and those with mental health issues may face additional obstacles. A cooperative strategy that takes into account each person's preferences, goals, and potential roadblocks is necessary to overcome motivational barriers and promote adherence.

3. Physical Health Considerations- It is critical to address physical health issues, particularly when people are possibly managing co-occurring conditions. Exercise interventions are made safe and customized to meet the specific health needs of each patient through the collaborative efforts of mental health and medical professionals.

4. Resource Accessibility- The viability of exercise programs can be impacted by the accessibility of resources, such as expert advice, open spaces, and fitness centers. Promoting inclusivity requires recognizing and eliminating obstacles to resource availability.

The relationship between physical activity and mental health is complex, as we learn more about the landscape of exercise as a preventive and therapeutic tool. The upcoming chapters will delve into personal narratives, examining true tales of resilience and transformation motivated by the strong link between physical activity and mental health. These stories highlight the relationship's universality and serve as a catalyst for a movement to promote social change that recognizes the interdependence of mental and physical health.

Chapter VI
Overcoming Barriers to Exercise

When trying to use exercise's transformational power for mental health, people frequently run into a number of obstacles that make it difficult for them to engage in regular physical activity. This chapter examines the typical barriers to exercise engagement, offers practical solutions for problems like time restraints and low motivation, and highlights social and community-based programs that promote physical activity as a culture for mental health improvement.

Common Obstacles Preventing Individuals from Engaging in Regular Physical Activity

Developing successful strategies to overcome obstacles requires an understanding of the challenges that people encounter. Time restraints, a lack of drive, physical health issues, financial hardships, and the belief that exercise is boring or unpleasant are common barriers. Establishing a setting that is supportive of regular physical activity begins with recognizing and resolving these obstacles.

Strategies for Overcoming Barriers, Including Time Constraints and Motivation Issues

1. Time Constraints- In the rush of contemporary society, time is often an enormous challenge to exercise. Embracing brief, intense workouts, incorporating physical activity into everyday routines (e.g., walking or cycling to work), and prioritizing self-care by acknowledging the long-term mental health benefits of exercise are some strategies to overcome time constraints.

2. Motivation Issues- It can be difficult to stay motivated, particularly when under stress or in a bad mood. Motivation can be strengthened by establishing reasonable and doable goals, finding enjoyable ways to exercise, looking for social support, and applying positive reinforcement strategies. Furthermore, fostering a sustainable commitment to physical activity can be achieved by focusing on the intrinsic benefits of exercise, such as enhanced mood and general well-being, in order to cultivate an intrinsic motivation.

Community and Societal Initiatives to Promote Physical Activity for Mental Health

Recognizing that individual efforts are amplified within a supportive community, initiatives at the community and societal levels play a pivotal role in promoting physical activity for mental health.

1. **Community Fitness Programs-** People can participate in physical activity in a supportive setting by creating inclusive and accessible community fitness programs. These programs can include anything from outdoor activities that promote a sense of community and shared well-being to group exercise classes.

2. **Workplace Wellness Initiatives-** Employers can support mental health by introducing workplace wellness programs that promote physical exercise. This could involve setting aside time for exercise, offering fitness challenges, or setting up spaces that encourage movement while at work.

3. **Public Spaces and Urban Planning-** The accessibility of exercise opportunities is influenced by the way public spaces and urban environments are designed. A more physically active society is facilitated by the development of parks and recreational areas, the creation of pedestrian-friendly neighborhoods, and the incorporation of physical activity infrastructure into urban planning.

We create a culture where physical activity is valued and prioritized for mental health by addressing common obstacles, putting practical strategies into practice, and supporting community and societal initiatives. The chapters that follow will shed light on individual transformation tales, illustrating the various ways in which people have overcome obstacles, embraced physical activity, and seen improvements in their mental health. These stories are inspirational, highlighting the possibility for change that exists for everyone when the strong link between physical activity and mental health is acknowledged and accepted.

Chapter VII
Personal Stories of Transformation

Personal narratives become vivid threads in the complex tapestry of the relationship between exercise and mental health, telling tales of resiliency, success, and deep transformation. This chapter presents stories and anecdotes from people who have experienced the lowest points of mental illness and found comfort, empowerment, and rejuvenation in engaging in regular physical activity. We examine the variety of experiences that highlight the universality of the relationship between physical activity and mental health through these narratives.

Anecdotes and Narratives of Individuals who have Experienced Positive Mental Health Outcomes through Exercise

1. Finding Healing in Running- Sarah, a young professional successfully managed the challenges posed by panic attacks and anxiety. Sarah found comfort in running, where each step turned into a potent exercise in taking back control. Her feet tapping on the sidewalk had a steady beat that matched the slow return of her mental balance. Sarah found a renewed sense of strength and resilience through running, which also helped to lessen her symptoms of anxiety.

2. Weightlifting and Empowerment- Ben's path is one of empowerment and self-discovery. Ben, who struggled with low self-esteem and body image, turned to strength training for solace. He began to use lifting weights as a metaphor for the observable improvements in his body and mind. Ben's relationship with himself changed as a result of the discipline and focus needed in the weight room, which led to an increase in confidence and a positive self-image.

3. Yoga for Emotional Restoration- The central theme of Maria's narrative is the use of yoga as a tool for emotional healing. Maria, who was struggling with her past trauma, turned to the mat for comfort. She was able to reestablish a safe connection between her body and emotions through the purposeful movements and mindfulness that are inherent in yoga. Maria found a way to emotional healing as well as relief from the symptoms of post-traumatic stress disorder through this gentle practice.

Diversity of Experiences and the Universality of the Exercise-Mental Health Connection

The variety of these narratives highlights how exercise and mental health are universally linked. It is not limited by an individual's age, gender, cultural background, or particular mental health issues. The universality is found in the common human experience of embracing physical activity with intention in order to find resilience, empowerment, and hope.

1. Cultural Perspectives- These stories are made richer by the diversity of cultural viewpoints. Different cultures have different ways of incorporating physical activity into mental health practices, ranging from traditional dance as a form of expression to group activities that combine exercise and social interaction.

2. Age and Life Stages- Personal narratives cover a range of life stages, from seniors discovering new vitality in their golden years to teenagers navigating the tribulations of puberty. The relationship between exercise and mental health is a constant throughout life's many journeys.

3. Intersectionality and Inclusivity- The relationship between exercise and mental health is inclusive of people of all backgrounds, abilities, and orientations because it acknowledges the intersectionality of identities. These tales are woven with inclusivity, highlighting the fact that anyone can benefit from exercise's transformational potential.

Examining these individual accounts reveals the significant influence exercise has on mental health. These tales are sources of motivation, demonstrating that the relationship between physical activity and mental health is not a one-size-fits-all solution but rather an enduring example of the human spirit. In the final chapters, we will look at doable strategies for designing long-lasting workout regimens, stressing the value of flexibility, social support, and incorporating physical activity into various life stages and situations.

Chapter VIII
Creating a Sustainable Exercise Routine

Embarking on the journey of exercise for mental well-being is not merely a commitment to sporadic activity but a cultivation of sustainable habits. In this chapter, we explore practical strategies for seamlessly incorporating regular exercise into busy lifestyles, emphasizing the pivotal role of social support and accountability, and providing insights into adapting exercise to different life stages and circumstances.

Tips for Incorporating Regular Exercise into Busy Lifestyles

1. Prioritize and Schedule- Making time for exercise in the midst of everyday chaos demands deliberate prioritization. Set aside time for exercise sessions as non-negotiable appointments, giving them the same priority as other commitments or meetings at work.

2. Short, Intense Workouts- When you are pressed for time, choose shorter, more intense workouts. Exercises such as high-intensity interval training (HIIT) provide quick and easy methods to increase heart rate and improve mental health.

3. Incorporate Physical Activity into Daily Routines- Include physical activity in routine tasks by cycling or walking short distances, using the stairs instead of the elevator, and doing quick stretches when you have a break. Over the course of the day, these little bursts of movement add up to total physical activity.

The Role of Social Support and Accountability in Maintaining an Exercise Routine

1. Find a Workout Buddy- Having a workout partner offers motivation and support to one another in addition to a social element. Exercise becomes more enjoyable and accountable when it is shared.

2. Join Group Classes or Teams- Teams in sports or group classes foster a sense of unity and common objectives. Peer pressure encourages accountability, which increases the likelihood that people will stick to their fitness regimens.

3. Utilize Technology for Accountability- Leverage social media platforms that promote accountability, online communities, and fitness applications to fully embrace the digital age. Motivation can be increased by participating in challenges, sharing workout accomplishments, or getting online support.

Adapting Exercise to Different Life Stages and Circumstances:

1. Prenatal and Postnatal Exercise- Exercise must be adjusted for people going through pregnancy or the postpartum period. Exercise stays a supportive part of overall well-being during these life stages thanks to prenatal and postnatal fitness classes, modified workouts, and professional guidance.

2. Exercise in Midlife and Beyond- As people get older, their priorities may change to include activities that promote flexibility, balance, and joint health. Taking up exercises like yoga, walking, or swimming can help you stay fit overall and meet your body's changing needs.

3. Navigating Health Challenges- People with health issues can modify their exercise regimens to fit their unique needs. Exercise can be modified to accommodate health conditions and enhance wellbeing with the help of healthcare professionals and fitness experts.

It is clear from our exploration of the tactics for designing a sustainable workout regimen that adaptability, flexibility, and a positive atmosphere are essential components of success. In the last chapter, we summarize the main ideas covered, make a case for why integrating exercise into mental health treatment should be given top priority, and consider the possible outcomes of a culture that promotes and values both mental and physical health.

The Story of James on how he Created a Sustainable Exercise Routine

James's journey towards creating a sustainable exercise routine is a testament to the transformative power of commitment and resilience in the pursuit of both physical and mental well-being.

A few years ago, James found himself caught in the whirlwind of a demanding job, stress, and a sedentary lifestyle that took a toll on his mental health. Struggling with anxiety and feeling the weight of daily pressures, he realized that a change was necessary for both his body and mind.

Motivated by a desire for holistic health, James embarked on a mission to integrate exercise into his daily routine. Knowing that a sustainable approach was crucial for long-term success, he started small. Walking became his first step towards a healthier lifestyle. Each morning, he dedicated a few minutes to brisk walks, gradually increasing the duration as his stamina improved.

To maintain consistency, James identified activities he genuinely enjoyed. He experimented with various exercises, from cycling to yoga, until he found the perfect blend that resonated with him. This not only made the routine enjoyable but also ensured that he looked forward to each session.

Understanding the connection between physical activity and mental health, James experienced a positive shift in his mood and energy levels. Exercise became his sanctuary, a time to release stress and refocus his mind. He began to notice improvements in his concentration, sleep quality, and overall outlook on life.

James didn't stop there; he incorporated mindfulness practices into his routine, seamlessly weaving moments of meditation and gratitude into his post-exercise cool down. This holistic approach enhanced the mental health benefits of his physical activities.

Through consistent effort and a commitment to his well-being, James not only transformed his lifestyle but also discovered a newfound passion for promoting the connection between exercise and mental health. His journey serves as an inspiring example for others, demonstrating that sustainable habits can lead to a healthier, happier life.

James's story can inspire readers to embrace the journey towards holistic well-being, highlighting the transformative impact of a sustainable exercise routine on mental health.

The Story of Anne on how she Created a Sustainable Exercise Routine

Anne's story is a powerful testament to the life-changing impact of cultivating a sustainable exercise routine for the betterment of mental health.

In the midst of life's challenges, Anne found herself grappling with stress, anxiety, and a sense of overwhelm. Determined to reclaim control over her well-being, she embarked on a journey to integrate exercise into her daily life.

Understanding the importance of sustainability, Anne adopted a gradual approach. She started with simple exercises that aligned with her fitness level and gradually increased the intensity as her strength improved. Rather than succumbing to the pressure of a rigorous routine, she prioritized consistency over intensity.

To keep things engaging, Anne diversified her workouts. From invigorating morning walks to exploring dance-based fitness, she discovered activities that resonated with her passion and kept her motivated. This variety not only made exercise enjoyable but also ensured that she stayed committed in the long run.

Recognizing the synergy between physical and mental well-being, Anne used her exercise routine as a form of self-care. Whether it was a jog in the park or a calming yoga session, these moments became a sanctuary for her mind to unwind and rejuvenate. Anne observed a profound positive shift in her mood, experiencing a newfound sense of clarity and resilience in the face of life's challenges.

Anne's commitment extended beyond structured workouts; she embraced an active lifestyle. Choosing stairs over elevators and opting for outdoor activities with friends became integral parts of her routine. This holistic approach not only reinforced the mental health benefits but also made exercise seamlessly woven into her daily life.

As Anne's journey unfolded, she became an advocate for the profound connection between exercise and mental health. Her story serves as an inspiration, showcasing that sustainable habits, tailored to one's preferences, can be a transformative force.

Conclusion

As we come to the end of our journey through the complex tapestry of "The Connection Between Exercise and Mental Health," it is appropriate to consider the journey toward transformation we have undertaken. We've delved into the depths of mental health and seen firsthand the enormous benefits exercise can have on our bodies, minds, and lives. Now that change is imminent, it is necessary to condense our understanding into a strong call to action.

The tales we have come across during this investigation bear witness to the incredible force of transformation. There is no denying that exercise is more than just a physical activity—it is a powerful inducement for mental health, as demonstrated by the experiences of Maria, the woman who sought sanctuary in a yoga studio, and the innumerable others who found comfort in rhythmic breathing. Let these anecdotes serve as a hopeful echo as we close this chapter, reminding us that good change is achievable and that all it takes is one small step—or maybe just one stretch.

Our voyage has shed light on the complex dance between the body and the mind. The neurobiological symphony that is produced by each stride, stretch, and deliberate movement has been understood. The science is unquestionable: endorphin release, neurotransmitter modulation, and brain reshaping are not just physiological results, but also doors to mental toughness and emotional resilience. It serves as a reminder that our bodies and minds are intertwined, and that when we take care of one, the other grows.

As we investigated the connection between exercise and mental health, we faced the obstacles that frequently prevent people from adopting this beneficial relationship. Piece by piece, time restraints, motivation issues, and social expectations were destroyed. Personalized strategies, routines that fit individual preferences, and encouraging communities were the keys to getting past these challenges. Let us take these realizations forward as we come to an end, dismantling the barriers that keep us from reaping the enormous rewards of leading an active and conscious life.

Our investigation is only the beginning; it is not the end. Exercise and mental health are linked in a way that is ever-changing and requires a lifetime commitment to self-care. As we come to the end of this chapter, let us accept that exercise is an ongoing, sustainable investment in our health rather than a temporary solution. Whether it's the energizing strides of a jog, the rhythmic flow of yoga, or the strength-building exercises of resistance training, let the knowledge that every action, no matter how tiny, adds to our mental resilience to inform our decisions.

The knowledge gained from our investigation necessitates action—not just individually, but as a group. It's time to advocate for a wellness revolution, a change in society that acknowledges the relationship between mental and physical health. Let our neighborhoods be places where being healthy is a basic right rather than a luxury. Let's be change agents as we come to the end of this journey by supporting laws that give mental health first priority, schools that incorporate physical education into the curriculum, and workplaces that value employee well-being.

Finally, may "The Connection Between Exercise and Mental Health" serve as a roadmap, an inspiration, and a force for transformation. The journey continues in the decisions we make, the dialogues we encourage, and the communities we establish. May the realization of this deep connection serve as the spark for a more promising and health-conscious future for both people and societies. May we clear the path for a society in which seeking mental health is not only accepted but also embraced, and where the ripple effects of our efforts will contribute to a wellness symphony for future generations.

www.ingramcontent.com/pod-product-compliance
Lightning Source LLC
Chambersburg PA
CBHW060913260726
48661CB00008B/3622